£3.20

CW01151734

INTERMITTENT FASTING FOR WOMEN OVER 50

A Proven Step-By-Step Guide to Burn Fat, Delay Aging and Get Healthy. Boost Your Metabolism and Detox Your Body without Deprivation, Discover a New Lifestyle

GEENA MOORE

All Rights Reserved. No part of this publication may be reproduced in any form or by any means, including scanning, photocopying, or otherwise without prior written permission of the copyright holder. Copyright © 2020

DISCLAIMER

This book is meant for educational and information purposes only. It is not meant to give any medical advice, diagnose, or treat any medical conditions. No medical claims are made in this book. The nutritional advice given in this book will not treat or cure medical conditions, metabolic disorders, or other illnesses. The nutritional advice is meant for healthy individuals who want to improve their appearance for cosmetic reasons and not to treat illnesses of any kind.

You should always consult your physician or other healthcare provider should you have any questions regarding a medical condition or treatment plan.

The author is not a MD or RD and cannot be held liable or responsible to any person or entity with respect to any information contained in this book. The reader/user assumes all risks for any injury, loss or damage caused or alleged to be caused directly or indirectly by using the information contained in this book.

Table of Contents

Introduction 1

Chapter 1 - Positive Effects and Benefits of Intermittent Fasting 12

Chapter 2 - Detox your Body with Intermittent Fasting 22

Chapter 3 - Can the Intermittent Fasting Be good for you? 34

Chapter 4 - The Dos and Don'ts of Intermittent Fasting for 50+ Women 47

Chapter 5 - Fasting, Eating and Training: the Right Moves 52

Chapter 6 - Healthy Habits Increases the Efficacy of if for 50+ Woman 62

Chapter 7 - Main FAQ on Intermittent Fasting 72

Chapter 8 - Recipes of Intermittent Fasting 85

Conclusion 150

Introduction

Many people are drawn to intermittent fasting for the sole purpose of weight loss. It is a good thing, as we have been blindsided for too long by vague and complicated diet plans and exercise regimens that lead us nowhere in terms of weight loss and good health. This gets even more difficult by the fact that we have hardly any idea of what goes on in our bodies when we are following these so-called diets. But as we saw earlier, the processes occurring in our bodies are not to our advantage at all. We have also seen, in broad terms, how intermittent fasting helps us lose weight.

Our body, and every single cell in our body has an inherent intelligence that works toward keeping us healthy. Each cell is naturally programmed to function this way. All the healing, repair and restoration processes in our body are carried out by the help of this very inherent intelligence. But when we take a meal, the focus of the cell shifts from bettering the body conditions to digesting the partaken food. When we eat continuously for every six to eight hours, the focus is more or less always focused on digesting the meal. The body then doesn't function toward the repair and restoration purpose for which the cell intelligence was initially intended. Fasting deals with this issue. When we fast, the cell intelligence is free to concentrate its efforts on other useful processes that are necessary for cleansing and purification. As soon as the digestion of the previous meal is completed the cleansing process begins.

But even this is not as simple as it sounds. Understanding what truly occurs inside our body cells and arming ourselves with this knowledge will help us in handling our fasts better. Fasting for prolonged periods of time is not easy and having the knowledge of what is happening at the micro-level will be a great motivation to carry the fasts to completion.

For the sake of this let's consider a water fast of three days. This fast would mean that an individual partakes of a large meal and then goes without food for the next three days. What they take instead are calorie-free beverages and plain water. Creamed and sweetened coffee or flavored water are not allowed during the fast. To derive maximum benefit from the fast, and get the best optimum results, they stick to just one large meal, full of carbs, proteins, and fiber and simply make do with plain water for the rest of the three days. Now, even though we don't generally recommend the water fast, it is useful in terms of learning what happens in the body during a fast. If you decide to partake in a water fast, like that described above, we highly recommend that you only do so under strict medical supervision.

Start your fast with a slow fasting schedule. Begin with a 12/12 fast or 14/12 fast at the most. Let your body get used to the fasting concept before taking a plunge into deeper, more intense fasts.

1. Begin by choosing a style of intermittent fasting that you feel suits you best and that you are confident you can carry through.
2. Start your fast the previous night to ensure you have a safe start to your fast while you sleep. For example, if on the night before your fasting day, you have a good large meal at 8 pm, start your fast time after two hours from your meal. So you would start your fast at around 10pm.

3. For our example, let's assume you are fasting the 12 to 14-hour fast schedule. If you wake up in the morning at around 6 am, you have already completed more than half of the fast. You have only four to six more hours to go to complete your fast.
4. If you can engage yourself in light exercise or walking, or a bit of yoga, that could easily knock another hour off of your fast.
5. Get by with water or plain or herbal tea without sugar or cream.
6. By 10 am you will have successfully completed a 12hour fast and you would only need two more hours if a 14-hour fast was your plan. If 12 hours was your plan, then you can pat yourself on the back for an easy breeze through fast.

To stay in the game and see yourself through to the end of your fast can be a challenge at the beginning. Extreme hunger pangs, headache, and stomach aches can make it difficult as you start your fasts to keep going hour by hour. Use the following tips to keep ahead of your fasts, avoid weakness, and stay motivated.

Begin by keeping a journal of your fasting experience. Not everything you go through during your fast with dates. Include your fasting schedule, you're eating window hours, what you had in your meal, and what you intend to have during your fast.

Also, include any symptoms you might notice. Do you feel dizzy and woozy? Write that down. Are you feeling heartburn or stomach cramps? Note that down too, along with time. This will help you analyze your body's responses to the fast when you have everything written before you for easier comparisons. It will help you understand how many hours of the fast were symptom-free and what symptoms began after how many hours.

Intermittent fasting isn't a new fad. Fasting has been in practice since time immemorial. People have been fasting for as long as humans have lived for various reasons. Humans have fasted for medical, spiritual, and religious reasons for years. Almost all religions have a ritual of some kind of fasting. Yet, when people are first introduced to intermittent fasting, their first feeling is that of fear. Who would want to starve? But intermittent fasting isn't something to worry about.

What we do not realize is that even without a single true fast in our lives, we still have experienced fasting. Our first day of the meal is known as 'breakfast,' because we have been fasting all through the night. If you can realize this, then your intermittent fasts become much easier.

In our race toward good health and weight loss, we have passed through many doors none of which led us to our goal. Now that we know and realize what a gift intermittent fasting can be, we can hope to finally breathe in relief. Intermittent fasting when done right, can be a boon to our body.

Benefits of Intermittent Fasting for Women Over 50

Some health benefits of intermittent fasting for women over 50 include:

Activating Cellular Repair

Fasting has been known to kick start the body's natural cellular repair function, get rid of mature cells, improve longevity, and improve hormone function. All things that tend to take a battering as people age. This can alleviate joint and muscle aches as well as lower back pain. As the cells are being repaired and the damage is undone, it helps with the skin's elasticity and health too.

Increase Cognitive Function and Protects the Brain from Damage

Intermittent fasting may increase the levels of a brain hormone known as a brain-derived neurotrophic factor (BDNF). It may equally guard the brain against damage like a stroke or Alzheimer's disease as it promotes new nerve cell growth. It also increases cognitive function and could effectively defend a person against other neurodegenerative diseases as well.

Weight Loss

When people have belly fat, it can cause many health problems that are associated with various diseases as it indicates a person has visceral fat. Visceral fat is fat that goes deep into the abdominal surrounding the organs. Belly fat is terribly hard to lose, especially for an aging woman. Intermittent fasting has been known to help reduce not only weight but inches of over five percent of body fat in around twenty-two to twenty-five weeks (Barna, 2019).

Alleviates oxidative Stress and Inflammation

Oxidative stress is when the body has an imbalance of antioxidants as well as free radicals. This imbalance can cause both tissue and cell damage in overweight as well as aging people. It can also lead to various chronic illnesses like cancer, heart disease, diabetes, and also has an impact on the signs of aging. Oxidative stress can trigger the inflammation that causes these diseases.

Intermittent fasting can provide your system with a reboot, helping to alleviate oxidative stress and inflammation in a middle-aged woman. It also significantly reduces the risk of oxidative stress and inflammation for those overweight or obese.

Slow Down the Aging Process

As intermittent fasting gives both the metabolism and cellular repair a reboot it offers the potential to slow down aging. It may even prolong a person's lifespan by quite a few years especially if following a nutritious diet and exercise regime alongside intermittent fasting.

Intermittent fasting is an ideal lifestyle to follow while you are aging. It is a simple and effective way to put your body on the right track. You must never forget that the age will have its toll on the body. How your body will deal with it would depend upon your level of preparedness.

If you keep living a laid-back lifestyle waiting for the chronic diseases to have their toll, then there is nothing that can stop you. However, we all know how that pans out for most people.

Intermittent fasting can help you in improving most health biomarkers that ensure that you live a healthy and happy life.

The aging process is a natural phenomenon over which all living organisms have little or no control. As humans, however, we have the advantage of being able to plan a healthier lifestyle that will impact positively on our aging process, affording us the opportunity to make the most of our life after 50.

During the aging process, the ability your cells have to multiply and function normally begins to slow down. As a result, your skin, which is usually the first place women notice the signs of aging, begins to show tiny wrinkles and blemishes and may become quite dry.

The Science Behind Aging

Each person has a personal "pre-programmed" genetic code that governs their aging process. This is why some women look older than they really are (Heathman, 2020).

Your skin, the first area that indicates your age, and the single largest organ in your body, is exposed daily to pollution and free radicals (these are unstable atoms), both of which are believed to have a negative impact on aging.

Each atom requires a specific number of electrons for it to function. When an atom has insufficient electrons, it is known as a 'free radical.' It will try to join up (bond) with another atom to complete its electron count.

When oxygen atoms split into two, unpaired atoms, they become unstable free radicals that cause oxidative stress in your cells and body tissues. The unfortunate result of oxidative stress, which happens over a period of time, is not only a variety of illnesses but also the formation of wrinkles and possibly greying hair (Heathman, 2020).

Chapter 1 - Positive Effects and Benefits of Intermittent Fasting

Intermittent Fasting Affects the Role of Cells, Genes & Hormones

Many things occur in your body when you do not eat for quite a while. For instance, your body begins crucial processes of cellular repair and adjusts the hormone levels, so that contained body fat becomes more available. These are some of the changes that take place during the fast in your body:

1. Insulin levels: insulin levels drop dramatically in the blood, which promotes burning fat.

2. Human growth hormone: growth hormone blood levels can rise as much as five times as high. Increased levels of this hormone promote burning fat and building muscle and have several other advantages.

3. Cellular repair: Your body causes essential mechanisms of cellular repair, like cell waste removal.

4. Gene expression: A variety of genes & molecules have beneficial modifications in relation to survival and disease prevention.

Intermittent Fasting May Help you Lose the Weight as Well as Belly Fat

Most of those who attempt intermittent fasting do so to simply lose weight; intermittent fasting can help you consume fewer meals. If you make up for it by eating even more throughout the various meals, you may end up consuming fewer calories.

Intermittent Fasting May Decrease Insulin Resistance, Reducing your Possibility of Type 2 Diabetes

In recent decades, type 2 diabetes has now become extremely prevalent. Its key characteristic in terms of insulin resistance is higher blood sugar levels. Anything that increases insulin resistance would help reduce blood sugar levels as well as defend against type 2 diabetes. Curiously, intermittent fasting is shown to have major advantages for insulin resistance, contributing to a remarkable drop in blood sugar.

Intermittent Fasting May Reduce Oxidative Stress & Body Inflammation

One of its moves towards aging, as well as other chronic diseases, is oxidative stress. It includes unstable molecules, known as free radicals that react to and damage other essential molecules (such as protein and DNA). Many studies indicate that intermittent fasting can improve the body's oxidative stress resistance.

Intermittent Fasting Could Be Advantageous for Heart Health

Heart disease is the greatest killer in the world right now. It is understood that specific health indicators ("risk factors") are either associated with an enhanced or reduced risk of heart disease. Numerous specific risk factors like blood pressure, total plus LDL cholesterol, inflammatory markers also blood sugar levels have been shown to strengthen by intermittent fasting.

Intermittent Fasting Causes different Mechanisms for Cellular Repair

The body cells initiate a process of cellular "waste removal" called autophagy when we fast. It includes breaking down the cells and metabolizing the damaged and defective proteins that, over time, build up within the cells. Enhanced autophagy could provide defense against a variety of illnesses, including cancer, as well as Alzheimer's.

Intermittent Fasting Can Help Prevent Cancer

Cancer is a horrible disease that is defined by uncontrolled cell growth. Fasting is shown to have some positive effects on metabolism, which may contribute to reduced cancer risk. Despite the need for human studies, promising indications from animal studies suggests that intermittent fasting can help to prevent cancer.

Intermittent Fasting Is Helpful for your Brain

Sometimes, what is beneficial to the body is good for the brain too. Intermittent fasting enhances the different metabolic features that are considered to be critical for brain health. It involves lowered oxidative stress, decreased inflammation, and decreased levels of blood sugar as well as insulin resistance. Several rat studies have also shown that intermittent fasting can stimulate the development of new nerve cells, which will improve brain function.

Intermittent Fasting Can Help with Alzheimer's Disease Prevention

Alzheimer's disease is the most prevalent neurodegenerative illness in the world. There is no treatment available regarding Alzheimer's, and it is important to prevent it from occurring. A rat study shows intermittent fasting can postpone the emergence of Alzheimer's disease or decrease its severity. Animal studies also show that fasting will defend against all other neurodegenerative disorders, including disease caused by Parkinson & Huntington. There is still a need for further human research.

Intermittent Fasting Can Increase your Lifespan, Letting you Live longer

Some of the intermittent fasting's most promising uses may be its potential to prolong lifespan. Studies in rats have also shown that IF increases lifespan in a similar manner to constant restriction of calories. These variations in hormones, gene expression & cell function are linked to many of the advantages of intermittent fasting.

History of Intermittent Fasting

For spiritual or religious reasons, fasting has been part of human traditions since prehistory. In fact, it is mentioned in many of the world's sacred books: the Upanishad, the Mahabharata, the Bible (both in the Old Testament and in the New Testament), the Talmud, the Koran and the Book of Mormon.

But in reality, fasting itself is something that the human body is adapted from the beginning of its history. Because imagine that our ancestors did not have a refrigerator to store their food, and did not even know when they would hunt prey.

Then, the body is prepared to withstand a few days without eating food. Of course, with health consequences, but at least, keeping us alive.

Based on that, numerous studies have been carried out, which have now discovered that by controlling the hours and / or days of fasting, this could become a powerful tool.

It could be summed up by saying that intermittent fasting is the performance of regular fasting and feeding cycles in a controlled manner to obtain certain benefits.

According to different studies, the body does not decrease its metabolic rate until about 60 hours after fasting has begun. In fact, in the first 48 hours, the metabolism increases by up to 3.6%.

What Does this all Mean?

Well, the human body can spend up to 48 hours without eating food and with an accelerated metabolism (which would help burn calories). This makes sense if we think about it evolutionarily. Faced with food shortages, the body becomes alert: it increases the metabolism and tries to get all its strength to be able to get the necessary food.

If it does not succeed, it finally enters "survival mode." That is why, if we spent many days without trying a snack, our body would begin a process by which the vital organs would have priority. The body focuses on the heart beating and we can continue breathing, but gradually "abandons" other functions and slows the metabolism to the maximum.

With this in mind, intermittent and controlled fasting can have many health benefits. Well, at the time of fasting when the metabolism increases, we will lose weight first. But we can also benefit from other aspects.

Intermittent Fasting Is Spiritual

We had already heard about intermittent fasting, inquiring more about the spiritual process of Buddhism. This explains that fasting is a very powerful purification practice.

It is usually done during the fourth Tibetan month, the full moon day that celebrates the birth and illumination of the dearest Buddha. In Asia, we had the opportunity for monks to tell us that, by practicing fasting with this intention, positive actions in your life are multiplied by ten million. They practice it in that month and on many other occasions of the year for different reasons.

Logically, the monks do not do it to lose weight, but to meditate and have greater concentration and attention of the present moment. Since if you are doing digestion or thinking about food it will be much harder to concentrate.

They also practice it as a technique of detachment from matter, understanding that eating is a pleasure invented by man. In this way, we could all have a healthy relationship with food.

We loved to see how they meditated for compassion for others. An act completely devoid of selfishness. However, when it comes to doing something for others, we always find obstacles to not putting anything into practice.

Lack of time is the favorite excuse, economic problems, the society in which we live, the acceptance of the people around us, etc.

All this happens because our mind is undermined by negative programming of the past. The good news is that these schedules can be erased by doing purification practices such as fasting.

Chapter 2 - Detox your Body with Intermittent Fasting

Your body is a magnificent piece of creative magic that was built to operate for the entire length of your life on earth. It is made up of a number of complex systems, each of which has a vital role to play in sustaining your life. When any one of these systems is compromised in any way, the negative knock-on effect for the entire body can be devastating.

As you age, inflammation often becomes a challenge. The best way to rid yourself of the discomfits this brings is to embark on a good detox program. Start by taking stock of the type of food you are currently eating that may be causing inflammation. Plan to your diet to exclude as many of these foods as possible:

- **Refined sugar:** This is found in cakes, candy, sugar, and desserts.
- **Refined carbohydrates:** This is found in bread, pasta, pastries, and cookies.
- **Processed meats:** Some are ham, salami, bacon, and jerky

- **Foods with MSG:** Some foods are instant noodles, instant mash, etc.
- **Artificial trans-fats:** This can be found in certain margarine, french fries, fast foods, microwave popcorn, etc.
- **Alcohol.**
- **Vegetable and seed oils:** Some include soy, sunflower seed oil, etc.

Include a wide variety of anti-inflammatory foods such as broccoli, fresh vegetables, fruits, lean meat, fish, and lots of water.

The process of detoxification takes time. It is certainly not a 'quick fix' to your weight problem. However, if you embark on a detox program, choose one that is likely to sustain weight loss when the program ends. Many of the detox systems advertised are short-term solutions that encourage you to continue using their products indefinitely.

The Process of Detoxification

Detoxification is a normal, continuous, natural process whereby dangerous, potentially poisonous substances are removed from your body via your liver. Your kidneys, lungs, and colon also act to remove waste materials as does your skin.

The role of your liver is vital to your continued health and well-being. Once the liver becomes overwhelmed by toxins, it loses its ability to function optimally. Your liver is further compromised when you imbibe on a regular basis. The results are usually devastating for your body.

Many toxins are fat-soluble adding to your weight and generally poor health. They are difficult to break down and can continue to accumulate in your system leading to type 2 diabetes, coronary heart disease, and obesity to name but a few of the problems they cause.

The true Value of Detoxing for Women Over 50

Your body stores a large number of toxic substances that you have unknowingly ingested over a period of time. Preservatives, MSG, added flavoring, hormones in meat and dairy products, chemical residue from sprays used on fruits and veggies all too often go unnoticed and are consumed without awareness. Many of these chemicals inhibit weight loss by effectively 'blocking' your body's natural detox pathways.

When your liver is unable to cope with the overload of toxins in your body, an imbalance exists, and you become ill. You may suffer from a bloated sensation or your body may retain fluid and certain parts of your body, usually, your extremities may become puffy and swollen. Under these circumstances, detoxing may be worth considering to right the wrongs as soon as possible and get your body back on track to good health and optimum functionality.

To assist your body in ridding itself of these toxic substances, you need to start with a healthy diet that bolsters the ongoing detoxification process. Like any form of house cleaning which needs to be done regularly to be effective, your body also needs to cleanse itself constantly to be able to function properly.

Sufficient restful sleep is also vitally important as it is during periods of rest that your body has the chance to regenerate and repair itself.

Regular aerobic exercises go a long way to support detoxifying your body by improving your breathing, building muscles, and improving your fitness levels.

If your gut has sufficient healthy flora, it is able to cope better with the digestive process, thus ensuring you receive adequate nutrients. This also predisposes you to fewer inflammatory diseases and is likely to stave off the development of dementia.

In a perfect world, if your body is healthy and functioning well it will detoxify itself within four to eight hours, without any fuss or fanfare. However, it is likely that you are suffering from the effects of the toxic environment in which you live, work, and relax. If this is the case, you need to add support to assist your body with its detoxing program.

Support your Body in the following Ways

To encourage and support your body to rid itself of waste, you may need to consider the following:

1. Eat fewer, smaller meals,
2. Allow four to eight hours between meals,

3. Choose healthy, natural, organic foods where possible,
4. Eat more raw foods,
5. Keep yourself well hydrated,
6. Avoid the use of chemicals in your home and garden,
7. Read and educate yourself about maintaining a toxin-free environment,
8. Make use of chemical-free cosmetics,
9. Use water and air filters, and
10. Minimize your carbon footprint.

The more sustainable you are able to make your environment, the healthier you are likely to be and the slower you will age.

If you follow a healthy lifestyle and diet, there should be no reason for you to consider detoxing because your healthy liver does the job for you.

However, if this is not the case, or should you wish to lose some excess weight, you may benefit from embarking on a weight loss program. Bear in mind, that for any weight loss program to be fully successful, you should consider detoxing before you begin the program.

If your intention is to lose weight and get your body back into shape, you also need to commit to consistently following the program until you reach your goal weight. Thereafter, you should work at maintaining your goal weight.

So, overall, weight loss and detoxing don't just happen overnight. There is no quick fix and any diet or detox program promising you one should be viewed with suspicion.

To support and assist your body's natural daily detox routine carried out by the liver you may consider a detox diet that lasts no longer than three days. Continuous deep detoxing for lengthy periods can be more harmful to your health in that your body loses valuable proteins, minerals, vitamins, and water during a detox program.

A good starting point for detoxifying your body is to restrict your diet to fruit and veggies for a day or two. Thereafter, you may introduce lean meat. Cut out all fizzy drinks, alcohol, desserts, chocolates, and sugar in your coffee or tea. Cut down and gradually restrict all starches.

Potential Benefits Intermittent Fasting

Not only does intermittent fasting benefit your waistline, but it can also reduce the possibility of developing several dangerous diseases.

Heart health

Heart-heart failure is the world's main cause of death. High LDL cholesterol, high blood pressure and higher concentrations of triglycerides are among the top risk factors for heart disease development. One test of 16 obese women and men has demonstrated intermittent fasting in only eight weeks to reduce blood pressure by 6 percent. It was also found in a similar study that intermittent fasting reduced triglycerides by 32% LDL and cholesterol by 25%.There is no clear proof of the correlation between intermittent fasting and increased triglyceride rates and LDL cholesterol

Research of forty normal-weight individuals showed that 4 weeks of prolonged fasting during Ramadan's Islamic holiday did not contribute to a decrease of triglycerides or LDL cholesterol. Higher-quality trials with more rigorous methodology are required until researchers can better explain the impact on cardiac safety of intermittent fasting.

Diabetes

Intermittent fasting will also help to better control and raising diabetes risk.

Similar to constant caloric control, intermittent fasting seems to diminish some of the diabetes risk factors. It does this mainly by raising insulin rates and insulin tolerance. 6 months of intermittent fasting decreased insulin rates by 29 percent and insulin tolerance by 19 percent in a randomized controlled trial involving more than a hundred obese people. Rates of blood sugar stayed similar. Moreover, in individuals with pre-diabetes, 8 to 12 weeks of intermittent fasting have been proved to lower blood sugar levels by 3 to 6 percent and levels of insulin by 20 to 31 percent, a state in which levels of blood sugar are increased but not high enough for diagnosis. Intermittent fasting, though, cannot be as effective in terms of blood sugar for women as well as for men.

A study showed that control of blood sugar aggravated for females after 22 days of alternate-day fasting, whereas no bad effect on men's blood sugar was seen. In spite of this side effect, a decrease in insulin and its tolerance will possibly also decrease the possibility of diabetes, specifically for pre-diabetes individuals.

Weight Loss

When done properly, intermittent fasting can be a relatively easy way of losing weight, as regular fasts may assist you to eat fewer calories and shed pounds.

A variety of reports show that intermittent fasting is as successful for a short period of weight reduction as conventional calorie-restricted diets. A 2018 analysis of the research showed prolonged fasting in bulky adults resulted in an overall weight reduction of 15 lbs (i.e 6.8 kg) for over 3 to 12 months. Another study found prolonged fasting in overweight individuals for a span of 3 to 24 weeks decreased body weight by 3–8 percent. The study also showed that during the same span, participants decreased their waist perimeter by 3 to 7 percent. It must be remembered that the long-lasting effects of extended fasting on women's weight reduction continue to be seen.

Intermittent starvation tends to help in weight reduction in the short term. The amount that you lose, however, will probably depend on how many calories you ingest in non-fasting days and how long you conform to the living style.

A variety of experiments on humans and animals indicate that prolonged fasting may often offer certain health benefits.

Reduced Inflammation

Few studies have found that intermittent fasting can lower-key inflammatory markers. Chronic inflammation can give rise to weight and numerous health issues.

Enhanced psychological health

Another study showed those 8 weeks of intermittent fasting reduced binge eating and depression actions in obese adults while refining body image.

Improved Longevity

Intermittent fasting was found to extend the lifetime by 33 to 83 percent in rats and mice. There has yet to be known the impact on the human lifespan.

Reserve Muscle Mass

This fasting tends to be more successful than constant calorie restriction in maintaining muscle mass. Also at rest, high muscle mass makes you eat more calories. Especially, the health effects of extended fasting for women in well-made clinical trials must be investigated more thoroughly before any conclusions are taken.

Chapter 3 - Can the Intermittent Fasting Be good for you?

This is one of the first questions that arises in the mind when trying to begin anything new. This question is natural and important. Before anyone else, you must feel completely satisfied and convinced with the idea or maintaining it for the long-run would become extremely difficult.

However, a better question would be:

Why Do you Need to Do anything?

This is a question that crosses the mind of every person who is in the process of transition. However, for women entering into their 50s, this question becomes all the more important. The importance of this question lies in the fact that your body is going through a lot of biological and hormonal changes. These are changes that can disrupt many things.

Menopause

This is one of the biggest changes that come as women enter their 50s. All women don't have menopause as soon as they reach 50. Some can have it early, while others may start experiencing it with time.

Menopause is not a small change. There is a whole biological process that stops once you reach a certain age, and the body takes time to adjust to those changes.

As a result, several issues can arise:

1. Sleep disorders or sleep apnoea
2. Sudden acne outbreaks
3. Tummy discomfort
4. Change in appetite
5. Brain fog and unexplained fatigue
6. Mood swings

Vaginal Dryness and poor Sex Drive

Some of these may look like common symptoms, but if you are not proactive in your life, these issues can take a toll on your life.

Obesity

This is another big issue that comes to haunt women once they start advancing in age. As you age, the chronic effect of poor diet, bad eating habits, and unhealthy lifestyles start to take control of your body. Youth is very powerful; it has a big capacity to consume energy, but as you age, your capacity to burn calories goes down and obesity becomes a huge problem. Many people look at obesity as primarily a cosmetic issue and then a metabolic issue. They are wrong. Obesity is a metabolic issue and it can become a big health hazard.

It never comes alone. It brings with itself metabolic disorders like diabetes, high blood pressure, heart problems, PCOS, and several other such problems.

Chronic Illnesses

Chronic conditions don't develop overnight. They keep simmering inside your body and when you are at your lowest point; when your immunity is weak; when your lifestyle is inactive, they start showing their effect. The time after the 50s is the fit time for that.

These are very strong reasons that you need to do something so that you don't fall into the trap of these problems. The more active your lifestyle is, the stronger your immunity is; the more reasonable your weight is, the better will be your health and your life ahead.

The 50s is not the final destination; it is the transit station. It is the stage when you are entering into a new phase of life and getting accustomed to new realities. At this stage, one really can't expect to bring drastic changes in life. Making even small changes is so difficult as so much is happening in life.

This is the reason Intermittent Fasting is the best because it can help you with all these issues, and it doesn't even require any significant change in the lifestyle that's very difficult to bring.

1. Intermittent fasting will help you in dealing with the changes that are coming due to menopause. It will improve your lifestyle for better, and hence menopause wouldn't be able to do much damage.
2. Intermittent fasting is one of the best ways to control obesity. It has become a craze because the effect of Intermittent Fasting on fat burning is

amazing. Hence, by following intermittent fasting, you will be able to manage your weight easily.

3. Most of the chronic illnesses are somewhere related to your diet and lifestyle. Intermittent fasting can help you in improving both, and hence the risk of chronic illness also goes down.

Therefore, intermittent fasting is definitely a boon for you if you can incorporate it into your life. It is good for anyone who is already not fighting some serious health condition or an eating disorder.

In case you fall in the following categories, intermittent fasting is a healthy lifestyle change:

1. A woman with a serious eating disorder
2. A woman suffering from anorexia or bulimia
3. Diabetic
4. Pregnant

Highly underweight

Women suffering from diabetes, high blood pressure, PCOS, and serious heart conditions must consult their physician before starting intermittent fasting as fasting can cause rapid changes in the blood sugar levels.

Hence, a dose adjustment and close monitoring may be required.

If you need to take medication for some chronic condition at short intervals, then also you must consult your physician before beginning intermittent fasting as several adjustments may be required.

Apart from that, if you are an otherwise healthy woman who wants to stay healthy and free from chronic health disorders, you can begin intermittent fasting, and it will have a wonderful effect on your mind, body, and soul.

Who Should and who Should Not Practice Intermittent Fasting (IF)

This could sound technical. But all it really means is to go without eating for extended periods.

Why would anyone want to? Okay, increasing numbers of fitness practitioners suggest that the exercise will help people lose their weight and improve their health. In reality, every day we do some sort of it. We call it inactive.

That's right. That's right. It could be described as a "fasting" interval, from the last meal in the night until the first meal you eat on the next day.(The time from the first meal to the last meal of your day can be called a "feeding" interval.) Therefore, try not to get too entangled in terminology.

Basically, people who decide to do intermittent fasting actually extend the time they don't eat. Everybody is, of course, jockeying "to get it right." It means that there are many different guidelines— Eat Stop Eat, Lean gains, Warrior Diet, 5:2 diet and more---all of which are going to cut down the "eating" window in one way or another and extend the "not eating" range.

Who Shouldn't Fast Intermittently?

Although intermittent fasting is healthy, it is not a form of diet that we can all use. First and foremost, please speak to an advisor regarding intermittent fasting, particularly if you have identified medical problems before beginning your routine. If you're unclear whether intermittent fasting is appropriate for you, this list might point out explanations for maybe not doing it.

People with Eating Disorders

If you have an eating disorder or previously had an eating disorder, it could be safer to stop intermittent fasting. Anyone with eating disorders may have an obsessiveness with dieting, and it may be attributed to psychological factors and not anything that is physiologically wrong with you.

Diabetics

While intermittent fasting decreases insulin and can be helpful to those who avoid diabetes, in certain situations, it may not be a successful approach. If you do have diabetes, it's better to speak to the doctor because the variations in type 1 diabetes and type 2 diabetes in your particular case may mean that you don't have the correct intermittent fasting.

Serious Fitness Fanatics and Athletes

What if you're committed to a rigorous workout schedule already? Intermittent fasting will help you — and it can potentially hinder your success too. Athletes require calories, and their bodies are now functioning to lose fat and to strengthen their muscles. This intensity enables nutrition to be a huge factor in their success; through rest and good eating, they seek to cure their bodies, looking at their nutrients, not just calories. Athletes seem to use more calories, of course, than the normal individual who is not as active. Although intermittent fasting is achievable on a strict exercise schedule, proper planning is necessary to ensure that the body isn't overworking.

People who Have Issues with Digestion

As if digestive problems were not too complicated to contend with on their own, introducing a wonky eating routine to the equation will just create further gastrointestinal discomfort. "If you have digestive issues (e.g., IBS), intermittent fasting can worsen the symptoms, or may even intensify digestive problems due to extended fasting bouts." Fasting cycles can interrupt the usual digestive system function, causing constipation, indigestion, and bloating. Gastrointestinal discomfort may be induced by consuming large meals – sometimes needed for IF forms that call for long-term fasting. "This is especially troubling for those with IBS who also have a more sensitive gut.

Nutrition, Concentration, and Motivation Are critical to everyday Activities

Food gives sustenance and strength that helps you to concentrate. When you're incredibly hungry, what you can think about is food that distracts the mind from the actual tasks at hand. If you have the sort of job or are involved in sports where strength and focus are required, intermittent fasting might not be appropriate for you.

Pregnant or Breastfeeding Women

Involving in it during pregnancy or breastfeeding may pose a risk to a child's health.

Pregnancy and breastfeeding need sufficient calorie consumption for the proper development of baby and milk productivity. Fasting cycles will mess with your food consumption, so breastfeeding and pregnant women shouldn't do intermittent fasting. "If you're attempting to get pregnant, IF may not be the diet of preference for you either. IF can even be related to fertility problems, triggering menstrual shifts, metabolic disturbances, and even early menopause in women.

People on Medications that Have to Be Taken with Food

These are several medicines that need to be consumed in the presence of food because without it, among many other side effects, they can render you feel nauseated or light-headed. Also, individuals who take a number of vitamins or nutrients per day may be impacted by IF fasting periods. For example, people who have a low blood iron count or anemia may need to take a daily iron supplement (or several) to help recover iron levels. Iron supplements are known for inducing diarrhea and can help alleviate the sensation when consuming them with meals. The moment you take an iron supplement can be adjustable, but what if you are on a medication that needs to be administered with food and at a very particular time of the day? That's where things get a bit messy because, in the end, getting into this diet is probably not a smart choice if it doesn't fit for the medications.

Those with a weak immune System or Have Cancer

Anyone that has undergone a significant illness previously, or are actually battling one, do not indulge in IF after first talking things up with a specialist. Here's why: "In most situations, sufficient calorie consumption is required to sustain lean body mass and a stable immune system that is vital for people with cancer or compromised immune systems," All people will speak to a specialist before trying intermittent fasting.

The Lifestyle Cannot Tolerate the Hours you Eat

Your job life will have a major effect on the willingness to participate in IF effectively. For instance, if you work the night shift and have to sleep in the afternoon because one of your feeding cycles comes in the afternoon, what do you do? Or worst, what if any of the fast happens when you are busy at work. Or, what if you work each day in various shifts and never have a regular schedule? Fasting cycles can trigger you to feel cold, with headaches and mood fluctuations. Having to deal with all those possible side effects could distract you from work and render you less efficient.

Chapter 4 - The Dos and Don'ts of Intermittent Fasting for 50+ Women

The Dos

Dos of Intermittent Fasting requires that these steps be followed to make full use of it.

- Daily contact with your doctor is an essential part of intermittent fasting. Try always to follow your doctor's suggestions and avoid using your own ideas, which can lead to harmful side effects.

- Plan your fast schedule those who do not plan will fail. Choose an appropriate time from your daily routine to work intermittently quickly. The best way to plan an irregular schedule is to consult a physician.

- Ask your doctor to analyze your body weight and calorie intake so that you can suggest the correct fasting plan.

- Try to follow your doctor's diet plan during eating hours and avoid taking calorie-enriched food. You don't want to become a cactus! Stay Hydrated

- Make sure you continue to drink water while limiting your calorie intake. Drinking water will cleanse your body and cleanse the blood vessels.

- If you cannot drink water in sufficient quantities, for some reason, try to take fruits and their juices which contain a large amount of water, such as orange and watermelon. Apart from water, tea, black coffee and natural juice, these are good add-ons to keep you hydrated.

Monitor your Body's Responses

- Check your body's circumstances closely. Try to track your body weight on a weekly basis and this will help you make a comparison and take decisions accordingly. Many people feel uncomfortable and tired when they first try intermediate fasting.

- Just make sure you don't lose weight by over-doing it. You probably know someone who started to do intermediate fasting and then became anorexic.

- Intermittently quickly to the degree that you could comfortably complete your daily work.

- Taking Vitamins Intermittent quickly will cause your body to have reduced vitamins. Taking the extra vitamins at the recommendation of the doctor to prevent this disease. Eat fruits that have large amounts of vitamins and minerals together with supplements. Avoid products that are artificially sweetened.

- Relax and enjoy the fun. It is hard for a person to spend time dreaming about all the donuts or hamburgers they will eat during an irregular holiday. It can lead to irritation, stress and depression sometimes. Avoid this by taking part in fun activities and talking to your friends. Try not to be alone and bored with quickness. It ought to be a happy time.

The Don'ts

To optimize the intermittent fast effect, stay away from the things below.

- Do not take too much before fasting. According to experts, heavy meals before fasting is strongly discouraged. It can harm your health, especially your stomach, due to the slow-burning nutrition in heavy or oily food.

- Always try taking the medium protein meal and low calories before fasting. At night you have natural sugar fruits, such as apple, mango, sweet melon, etc. Don't push too hard. Do not give your body priority over intermittent fasting if you feel ill or excessively exhausted at fasting.

- Experts warn against fasting in conditions of health such as diabetes, cancer and pregnancy. These conditions must be followed by precise steps. Consultation with a doctor is important for people with these health situations.

- Be not stressed out. Be calm and cool. Be stressed out. Stress can increase your body's cholesterol level. Fasting is not necessary if excessive stress levels are induced in the body. Yoga and deep breathing are good practices for stress relief.

- Don't do hard workouts such as yoga and jogging is always recommended to do during fasting. Remember that in the fasting state your energy level is lower. It goes without saying, therefore, that in this state you don't want to lift too much weight or run a marathon. Be comfortable for lighter workout.

Chapter 5 - Fasting, Eating and Training: the Right Moves

There are a variety of ways to actually do intermittent fasting, but the simplest and most common methods include taking advantage of your normal overnight fast by missing breakfast and moving forward a number of hours on the first meal of the day. Once you've passed the 12-hour mark from dinner the night before, you're in a much-fasted state and start relying on stored body fat for fuel.

The longer you remain in the fasted state, the stronger your fat change will likely get. Indeed, if you can hold this fasting for twenty to twenty-four hours, you can achieve an even greater amount of lipolysis and fat oxidation (fat burning in the mitochondria).

You can feel hungry and low-energy when you start with intermittent fasting first. In this case, it is suggested that beginning with baby steps, at first simply moving breakfast out for an hour or two, then gradually increasing the interval of fasting. As time goes by, and you are more adapted to fat, faster is easier. In those that are sedentary, this is the same as and exercises: at first, it is unpleasant and incredibly challenging, and then, once you are accustomed, it becomes simple and even fun.

Eat More Satiating Meals

The food you consume will have an effect on your ability to do, stick to your diet and stick to your fast, and that's where IF will help you out. Picture your normal diet on fat loss;

1. Morning bacon, or porridge
2. A quick lunch of unseasoned chicken breast, sweet potatoes and veggies followed
3. After your workout, add protein and water/milkshake
4. Then finish the day with an almost uninspiring evening meal

If you're fortunate, you can scrounge enough calories a couple of times a day to get a few handfuls of nuts. You're feeling unsatisfied and far from comfortable with the fact that you're going to have to do it all over again and again before you hit the weight of your target if you don't quit before then that's it.

Stay busy

The enemy is Boredom. It is the silent killer who comes in to slowly undo your momentum, breaking you down and dragging you backward. Only pause for a moment.

How many times hunger has driven you to eat more than you should, wish or even know that you are:

1. You do something boring at work, and the snacks let in the kitchen wake up.
2. You're watching Netflix at home, it's fine, just not captivating, and you're enjoying the snacks carelessly.
3. You're waiting for an airport flight and find you wandering the shops or sitting in the restaurants.

Yet what is the broadness the causes you to eat?

You should ask for dopamine, a chemical in the brain. Dopamine is the reason you feel good about reaching an objective and taking responsibility for reward-motivated behavior.

Ironically, eating will induce the release of dopamine and, as a result, the good feelings that it produces. More than that, it's junk food that makes you feel fantastic, particularly those high in sugar, fat and sodium!

This behavior can be seen in existing research showing that boring subjects consume more calories than non-bored subjects, with additional research showing "that boredom significantly increases both obese and average food consumption [subjects]."

It's really no wonder that you eat more when you get bored; you're practically hardwired to chase the high dopamine.

Blunt your Appetite

Hunger pangs would definitely set in from time to time when it is fasting. When this happens, the key is to counter your appetite, and the best way to do that is through 0 calorie drinks that help bring satiety and keep starvation in the bay until it's time to break your run.

Examples include beer, sparkling water, black coffee, black tea and green tea, and you're good to go as long as the drink is zero calories.

Untapped Brain

In a day, the average adult makes thousands of decisions, and hundreds are about food. This ultimately drains the brain of strength and motivation, which means less fuel needed to do better work for the innovative problem-solving. You have been painfully conscious of the benefits of taking fewer decisions every day. Particularly when it comes to very routine things, like what clothes you wear, where and when you do your job, and the kind and timing of the food you eat, of course. Instead of worrying about what's up for breakfast, you can get straight into your job and start using your brain that's untapped.

Impulse Control

For you, the shocking discovery in you maybe that how much you thought of reaching for a snack when you are working. This is particularly true when you didn't feel the work as engaging or enjoyable. You soon noticed the difference between your physiological appetite and your desire for Boredom. This realization not only helped you to improve your impulse control but also opened up a new dialogue inside you. In other aspects of your life, you started deciphering your emotional signals. That conscious lens taught you to turn up in a more successful way and to face your challenges. You notice that you have been more concerned with the various problems that you face in a day, and you are constantly searching for a more positive outlook on how you can manage them.

Break your Fast with a Daily Meal

Earlier, we touched on this when we talked about how it isn't an excuse to eat whatever you want. Like with every other diet out there, it only works for weight loss or muscle building if you maintain a calorie deficit or excess that is acceptable. This means you don't want to throw caution on the wind when it comes time to break your fast, particularly when your target is a fat loss.

Yeah, skipping breakfast releases calories to give you more space for your other meals, but if you're going to nuts, you'll erase the calorie deficit you've been working so hard to create. However, your meal size will depend on whether you have just worked out or are working out later in the day while breaking your fast.

Stick to a Routine

The Cambridge Dictionary describes the routine as a standard or fixed way of doing things and when it comes to How this can be done by; start and break the fast every day at regular times, use a weekly diet where you eat the same (or similar) things every day, and prepare food beforehand.

Getting a routine makes it easier to stick to your IF plan as you eliminate the uncertainty and second-guessing from the equation as you learn what works for you and stick to it daily. What you need to do is to follow through.

The Calories and Macros Fit

You'll finally get to the point where you make the wrong or easy option because you're worn out by decision makes muscle. By every the amount of choices you need to take each day, you eliminate the potential barriers to your success.

When you're struggling to make the change you want, and still find yourself straying from your diet and hours of fasting, you'll benefit from a regular implementation.

Give yourself Time to Adjust

Only wanting results right away, skipping the awkward novice phase and going straight to seasoned pro, or at least the 'I kind of know what I'm doing' part, is only natural. Saving the initial learning level, however, is setting you up to fail. You have to give yourself body time to adapt to fasting, particularly when it's your first time.

It's only normal to get hunger pangs on your first start and chances are you will mess up a few times too, that's fine and normal as well. It doesn't mean you have to give up or it isn't going to work for you. Rather, it's an opportunity to know, challenge why or how you messed up and take action to stop it from happening again.

Use the Right Mindset

If nothing else works for you, intermittent fasting is not a simple fix or workaround to meet your goals. It's yet another nutritional system that some people can function really well if used correctly and blends in with their lifestyle. Intermittent fasting produces amazing results, but these results depend on your reaching your calorie and macronutrient target, regularly training and applying progressive overloading.

The same applies to all diet setups, so you need to keep this in mind whether you are using IF or anything else. Here are three ways to help you take the attitude;

1. Set your goals on the basis of reasonable assumptions that what is actually possible was not possible what you wish
2. Be one-sided in your actions and recognize that the best path to success is a continuous commitment towards a particular target.
3. Be careful and know that just as you haven't lost the body of your dreams in a day, week or month, you won't create it that quickly.

Enjoy yourself

Intermittent fasting can have tremendous benefits in terms of dietary independence, and thus enjoyment, when done properly.

That is because you save yourself from 300-1,000 calories everywhere by missing breakfast, depending on what you usually consume.

You should then redistribute these calories to your lunch, dinner or 1 – 2 snacks to help you enjoy your diet more.

Chapter 6 - Healthy Habits Increases the Efficacy of if for 50+ Woman

Before you begin fasting, there are some things that you will want to do to prepare yourself. It may be difficult mentally and physically, especially if you are new to fasting. Your mindset will become very important as you are fasting, especially the longer you fast at one time. Getting yourself into the proper mindset before you begin will help you to stay focused while you are fasting.

Ensure you Are Fasting in a Healthy Way

When it comes to fasting, it is important to ensure that you approach it in a way that will be beneficial for our health, and that will not do more harm than good.

Firstly, you want to maintain flexibility with yourself and your body when fasting. If you are not feeling well as you are trying to fast, don't be afraid to eat a small amount on your fast days. This is especially true at the beginning when you first introduce fasting into your diet. If you try a water fast for example, and you feel lightheaded and weak, you may decide that you want to instead try an intermittent fasting method like 5:2 which would allow you to eat on your fast days, but in a greatly restricted amount. If you have your mindset on 24-hour water fast, then try the 5:2 method a few times before you try the full water fast in order to get your body comfortable with reduced amounts of food first.

Increase your Water Intake

As I mentioned, dehydration can accompany fasting since much of our water intake throughout the day comes from the food we eat, like fruits or vegetables. If you are feeling like you are dehydrated while fasting (dry mouth, headache), it is important to increase your water intake. You will also want to ensure you drink enough water each time you fast afterward. The recommendation is about two liters per day, but of course, this depends on your body size. In general, eight glasses of water that are about eight ounces each should give you enough water to be hydrated but when fasting, this must increase to about nine to thirteen glasses. This works out to be between two and three liters of water.

Pay Attention to your Body

If you are feeling very unwell while you are fasting, it is important to know when to stop fasting. It is normal to feel fatigued, hungry, and maybe irritable when you fast, but you may want to stop your fast if you feel completely unwell. In order to be safe, for your first few times fasting, keep the duration shorter, and work your way up to the desired amount of time. Also, keep some food on you in case you need to eat something due to low blood sugar or feeling unwell. Remember that you are fasting in order to take care of your body and your health and it should not make you feel worse.

Increase Protein Intake

Ensuring that you eat enough protein while fasting will have numerous benefits for you. Protein takes longer to digest, which means that the energy you get from protein will be longer lasting than the energy you get from other sources like carbohydrates- which is used up quite quickly. Eating enough protein will help to keep your hunger at bay, especially if you are doing the 5:2 method or a method where you will eat small amounts on your fasting days. This will keep you from having an energy "crash" similar to a sugar crash after you have quickly used up the sugars you have ingested.

Select the Foods you Eat Wisely

When you do break your fast or when you are eating small amounts on fasting days, choose the foods you eat wisely. You want to properly prepare your body to fast and keep it healthy while you do so. In addition to eating enough protein, you want to make sure that the other foods you eat are real, whole foods. Whole foods are those which are as close to those found in nature as possible. These are things like meats, vegetables, fruits, fish, eggs, and legumes. This will give you all of the nutrients you need to stay healthy. Eating fast food and processed foods on the days that you are not fasting will leave you feeling tired and without energy, especially if you are fasting the next day or have fasted the day before.

Consider Supplementation

Supplementing may be very beneficial and even necessary when fasting to maintain and improve health. Some essential nutrients and minerals that your body would greatly benefit from like Omega-3's or iron may be difficult to get in adequate amounts if you are fasting. For this reason, supplementing them may benefit you in terms of keeping you feeling healthy and energetic, as well as keeping your brain functioning to its full potential. You can take specific nutrients on their own in pill-form or you can opt for a multivitamin that will include all of the most essential vitamins and minerals for overall good health.

Avoid Over-Doing it in the Beginning

Keeping your exercise levels to a minimum while fasting is often necessary as your body will not have as many readily-available sugars or carbohydrates to provide you with the quick energy needed for a workout. This is especially important if you are beginning a fasting regimen for the first time. Your body will need time to adjust to fasting without being extra drained from working out as well. If you are planning to increase your levels of autophagy through a combination of fasting and exercise, wait until your body has adapted to your fasting routine before adding in the exercise portion of the plan.

When Not to Fast

There are times when fasting is not recommended for a person, no matter how used to fasting they may be. If your fasting day comes around and you are feeling any of the following symptoms, fasting that day will not be advisable for you. Knowing when to decide not to fast is important for your health and wellbeing.

If you are feeling sick, including nausea, diarrhea, and general feelings of sickness, take that day or the next few days off of fasting until you are feeling one hundred percent better. Your body needs all of the nutrition it can get while it is trying to fight off sickness and fasting will be taxing to the body, which will make it very difficult for it to fight off the illness.

Things to Take Note of to Ensure Success

Before you begin to fast, as with anything else you set out to do in life, it is important to be aware of your objectives and your motivations for doing it in the first place. It is unlikely that you are doing anything in life without a reason or a motivation for doing so, and if you think you are then maybe your objective is there in the back of your mind somewhere. Think about your objective before you begin, because when you are in the middle of your fast, you will need to look to that objective or motivation to keep you from changing your mind right then and there and breaking your fast for a doughnut.

The Biggest Obstacle: Your Mind

Everybody's objective will differ slightly and will likely be quite personal to them. Maybe you want to reduce your risk of cancer because it runs in your family. Maybe you have been obese for the majority of your life, and you are trying this as a means of weight loss and health improvement. Maybe you heard about it and challenged yourself to try it for a few months to see how it feels. Whatever your objective, writing it down will help to solidify it and make it real. Then, when you are wondering why on earth you decided to put yourself through this on the first day of your fast, you can look at that objective that you wrote down and it will re-inspire you to continue. When it comes to mindset, being aware of your motivation is extremely beneficial.

Your Expectations

By expecting that there will be some uncomfortable side-effects like hunger and irritability, you can greet them with the feeling of "Oh hello, I have been expecting you." Rather than "Oh no I am feeling so terrible what is going on?" If you are not surprised that you will feel a little bit uncomfortable while your body adapts to your fast, you will be able to greet it rather than fighting it, which will make you much more comfortable with it all.

It is important to recognize when fasting that this is a choice you are making for your health, your body or whatever specific objective you have. You must recognize that this is a choice you are consciously making and that you have decided to go through these times of fasting in order to later receive the benefits. If you lose sight of the fact that this is a choice you are making, you may begin to feel like a victim or like the universe is punishing you. This victim mindset will only make things harder for you. By taking responsibility for your decision to fast, you will not allow yourself to slip into this negative mindset and will instead feel confident and in control of your decision. This will help you to view things through the lens of appreciation rather than deprivation like I outlined above.

Your Emotions while Fasting

You can prepare as much as you like, but while you are fasting, you could meet some unexpected feelings. Challenging your body and mind often brings up many feelings for us, as it puts us in a state of self-reflection and deep thought. This is normal. Think about if you decided to run a marathon. While running, as your legs desperately want to give up and your body is tired, your mind will likely go to some deep places that they do not go when you are going about your regular daily duties. Fasting is similar to the marathon in this way as it can be very challenging for both the body and the mind.

When emotions come up during your fast, it is important to know what to do with them. The first step is to acknowledge them. By acknowledging these emotions, you can tap into them and examine them in more depth. The next step is to write them down. This can be a very quick note of how you are feeling or what the most challenging part is for you. By writing it down, you are processing this emotion and you are able to address it instead of pushing it away. When we push our emotions away, they do not really go away; they just go dormant for a short period of time only to come up later. By addressing them, you can examine what is going on inside of you.

Chapter 7 - Main FAQ on Intermittent Fasting

Question # 1: Can I Take Bone Broth?

First of all: what is bone broth - and why would anyone be interested in taking it?

In short, bone broth is the drink obtained by boiling the bones and connective tissue of different types of animals.

It is rich in vitamins, minerals, collagen, and other nutrients.

And it is precise because the bone broth is rich in nutrients that it becomes interesting for longer fasts.

Because it has the ability to replace nutrients (vitamins and minerals) lost during the fasting window.

After all, you are frequently eliminating water and minerals during this period through urine and perspiration.

Question # 2: What Breaks Fasting?

There is no single answer to this case - but calmly, let's explain it properly.

And by the end, you will understand the truth of why some people say that a certain food or drink "breaks" fasting, and why others say it does not.

In fact, the answer to that question is to distinguish between two types of fasting: insulin fasting and calorie fasting.

Insulin fasting

Insulin Fasting is a type of fasting where you will focus primarily on not raising your insulin.

That is, you will not be able to eat foods that raise insulin, being a little more permissive with foods that do not raise insulin.

And what are these foods that do not raise insulin?

Well, the only macronutrient that doesn't have much effect on insulin is fat.

Because both proteins and carbohydrates cause a certain increase in the levels of this hormone.

Question # 3: What Can I Eat Or Drink during Fasting?

As we said earlier, to reap the full benefits that intermittent fasting can provide, you simply shouldn't eat or drink anything that has calories.

On the other hand, we also argue that small amounts of good fats will not hinder your goals if you are only looking to control your insulin.

And finally, we also say that some authors defend the idea that eating very few calories (up to 50 kcal) would not break your fast - regardless of the source of those calories.

Even so, we know that some people prefer a summary list of foods to help them get started.

For this practical list helps to remember which foods and drinks can or cannot be consumed during the fast window - without necessarily "breaking your fast" or ending all its benefits.

For this reason, we have put down a short non-exhaustive list of foods that can be eaten without disturbing your fast.

Question # 4: But what about Sweetened Foods But No Calories? Like Coffee with Stevia, Erythritol or Sucralose, and even Zero Soda?

By now, you have understood that the idea of intermittent fasting is not to consume food - so as not to ingest calories, or to raise insulin.

So, using non-caloric sweeteners would be released, right?

Calm down - this issue is more complex than it may seem at first.

First, I strongly recommend that you understand the differences between the different types of low-carb sweeteners.

But, as we explained, even if we consider only sweeteners that do not raise insulin (as is the case with stevia, or even erythritol, for example), we still have an important question.

That (although this relationship is speculative - that is, unproven), there are possibly several potential mechanisms through which the use of sweeteners can interfere with metabolism.

And that even includes interactions with sweet taste receptors, which would stimulate other metabolic adaptations.

Certainly, more research is needed, but in our opinion, this is yet another sign that it can be smart not to abuse sweeteners.

And in our personal opinion, one thing is certain: the daily consumption of sweeteners is not ideal for your health - even though it may not hinder weight loss or break your fast.

Especially in the case of artificial sweeteners - and even more so in the case of zero soft drinks.

Question # 5: Who Can Do Intermittent Fasting?

An important question that people often have when we talk about fasting and its benefits is precisely who can and cannot fast (practice it).

The direct answer is that the practice of intermittent fasting is suitable for healthy adults.

It is even easier to speak who should not start fasting without first talking to their trusted doctor.

Question # 6: But Isn't Eating Right every 3 Hours?

Not really.

As we explained in our text "Eat every 3 hours" —"Do you still fall for that lie?""People adopt this practice for 4 alleged reasons."

That is, they think that eating every 3 hours will help them:

1. Speed up the metabolism,
2. Control blood glucose,

3. Control appetite,
4. Preserve your muscle mass.

However, these 4 points are controversial (not to say wrong) in the light of science - and eating every few hours may even make some of these results worse.

Again, if you want a more detailed explanation on this point, I recommend reading our full text on eating every 3 or 4 hours.

Question # 7: Does Fasting Slow Metabolism?

If you are paying attention to this text, you should already intuitively know the answer to that question.

No, intermittent fasting does not slow down metabolism.

The keyword in this sentence is "intermittent."

For it is clear that to spend very long periods (several and several days) without eating will imply a metabolic adaptation (that is, a slowing down of the metabolism).

Just as a very long and/or severe caloric restriction will also have the same effect.

This is because our body seeks to survive above all else.

So if you go without eating for several days, your body will seek to preserve energy.

However, on short fasts, our metabolism tends to increase.

In this case, one study found a 3.6% increase in metabolism on short fasts - and another study found that metabolism increased 10% during fasting.

This makes evolutionary sense: if our body seeks to feed, it needs to stimulate us, and not deprive us of the energy we have - so that we can hunt/collect food and thus obtain energy.

This is probably mediated by hormonal changes that occur during fasting, such as increased adrenaline.

Question # 8: Intermittent Fasting Causes Loss of Muscle Mass (Lean Mass)?

Another very common question is regarding the conservation of muscle mass when we practice fasting.

This question arises mainly because we always hear around (especially repeated as a mantra in gyms), that if you didn't eat every three hours, your body would start to burn muscles to provide you with energy.

Unfortunately, this is a very common myth - and we just have no idea where it came from.

If you read the question about "eating every 3 hours" that we answered above, then you understand that you don't have to eat every 3 hours to conserve your muscle mass.

On the other hand, you may be wondering if taking longer periods without eating (16, 24, 48 hours or more) would damage your lean mass.

But you can rest easy: during the fasting window, you will not break muscles as a form of energy.

In fact, your muscles can even serve as an energy source, but you have other reserves that are much easier for your body to use, such as fat in your belly and elsewhere, and glycogen.

Remembering that glycogen is our energy reserve in the form of carbohydrates, which is stored both in the liver and in the muscles, between the muscle cells.

Question # 9: Can I Exercise during Fasting?

Another very common question concerns fasting and physical exercise.

The most common questions are:

1. Can I train fasting?
2. Can I not eat anything after training?
3. Can I train fasting and continue fasting afterward?

Briefly, the answer to these questions and their variations is: you can do what you want.

You can train on a fast if you feel good, for example.

At the same time that there are people who are not feeling well, in which case they probably shouldn't be training fasting.

Of course, if you're on a high-carb, especially refined diet, eating every three hours; for a low-carb diet and still, start fasting and training hard, so it's normal that you don't feel well.

You need to give your body time to adapt to all these changes.

However, we believe that most people can, yes, train fasting after some time of adaptation, if they want to do so.

That is, there is nothing special about being fasting that prevents you from training.

You can even practice fasting and then fast for a few more hours until your lunch.

As we mentioned in the case of lean gains fasting, you don't necessarily need to have your first meal right before or right after your workout.

Question # 10: Which Supplements Do Not Break Intermittent Fasting?

Now that you know you can train on an empty stomach, without eating anything before and nothing afterward, maybe your next question is precisely related to supplements.

As we have said before, theoretically, fasting is a period when you should not eat anything.

However, there are exceptions, as in the case of insulin fasting.

So it is natural that doubts related to supplements arise as well.

Especially because there are supplements that do not really break the fast - because they do not contain calories.

Question # 11: What to Say When someone Criticizes your Fasting?

The truth is that, even with all the support that science gives to this practice, fasting is still a controversial topic for most people.

(As strange as it may be that we live in a society in which we skip meals occasionally and eat real food are controversial.)

So don't be alarmed if you receive unwanted criticism or comments from friends and family.

Chapter 8 - Recipes of Intermittent Fasting

Breakfast Recipes

1. Healthy Breakfast Smoothie

Preparation Time: 5 Minutes

Cooking Time: 1 Minute

Servings: 1

Ingredients:

- 1 ¼ cups coconut milk, or almond or regular dairy milk
- ½ cup kale or spinach, or both (¼ Cup each) if you prefer
- ½ avocado, sliced into smaller pieces
- ¾ cup cucumber, sliced into smaller pieces
- 1 cup of green grapes
- ¼ teaspoon ginger, peeled and grated
- 1 scoop Plant-based protein powder

- Honey to taste

Directions:

- Add all of these ingredients into your blender in the order they appear above.

- Blend them until the mixture is smooth

- Taste it and add as much honey as you desire

- Pour into a glass and serve.

Nutrition: Calories: 117, Fat: 15 grams, Protein: 20 grams, Carbs: 5 grams

2. Avocado Egg Bowls

Preparation Time: 10 minutes

Cooking Time: 40 minutes

Servings: 3

Ingredients:

- Coconut oil- 1 Teaspoon
- Organic, free-range eggs-2
- Salt and pepper- to sprinkle
- Large & ripe avocado- 1

For Garnishing:

- Chopped walnuts, as many as you like
- Balsamic Pearls
- Fresh thyme

Directions:

- Slice your avocado in two, then take out the pit and remove enough of the inside so that there is enough space inside to accommodate an entire egg.

- Cut off a little bit of the bottom of the avocado so that the avocado will sit upright as you place it on a stable surface.

- Open your eggs and put each of the yolks in a separate bowl or container. Place the egg whites in the same small bowl. Sprinkle some pepper and salt to the whites, according to your personal taste, then mix them well.

- Melt the coconut oil in a pan that has a lid that fits and put it on med-high.

- Put in the avocado boats, with the meaty side down on the pan, the skin side up and sauté them for approx. 35 seconds, or when they become darker in color.

- Turn them over, then add to the spaces inside, almost filling the inside with the whites of the eggs.

- Then, reduce the temperature and place the lid. Let them sit covered it for approx. 16 to 20 minutes until the whites are just about fully cooked.

- Gently add one yolk onto each of the avocados and keep cooking them for 4 to 5 minutes, just until they get to the point of cook you want them at.

- Move the avocados to a dish and add toppings to each of them using the walnuts, the balsamic pearls, or/and thyme.

Nutrition: Calories 215, Fat 18 grams, Carbs 8 grams, Fiber 2.6 grams, Protein 9 grams

3. Blueberries Breakfast Bowl

Preparation Time 35 minutes

Cooking Time: 0 minutes

Servings: 1

Ingredients:

- 1 teaspoon chia seeds
- 1 cup almond milk
- ¼ cup of fresh blueberries or fresh fruits
- 1 pack sweetener for taste

Directions:

- Mix the chia seeds with almond milk. Stir periodically.
- Place in the fridge to cool for 30 minutes, and then serve with fresh fruit. Enjoy!

Nutrition: Calories: 202, Fat: 16.8 grams, Protein: 10.2 grams, Carbs: 9.8 grams, Fiber: 5.8 grams

4. Feta-Filled Tomato-Topped Oldie Omelet

Preparation Time 5 minutes

Cooking Time: 6 minutes

Servings: 1

Ingredients:

- 1 tablespoon coconut oil
- 2 pcs eggs
- 1½ tablespoon milk
- A dash of salt and pepper
- ¼ cup tomatoes, sliced into cubes
- 2 tablespoons feta cheese, crumbled

Directions:

- Beat the eggs with the pepper, salt, milk, and the remaining spices.
- Pour the mixture into a heated pan with coconut oil.
- Stir in the tomatoes and cheese. Cook for 6 minutes or until the cheese melts.

Nutrition: Calories: 335, Fat: 28.4 grams, Protein: 16.2 grams, Carbs: 4.5 grams, Fiber: 0.8 grams

5. Carrot Breakfast Salad

Preparation Time: 5 minutes

Cooking Time: 4 hours

Servings: 4

Ingredients:

- 2 tablespoons olive oil
- 2 pounds baby carrots, peeled and halved
- 3 garlic cloves, minced
- 2 yellow onions, chopped
- ½ cup vegetable stock
- 1/3 cup tomatoes, crushed
- A pinch of salt and black pepper

Directions:

- In your slow cooker, combine all the ingredients, cover and cook on high for 4 hours.
- Divide into bowls and serve for breakfast.

Nutrition: Calories: 437, Protein: 2.39 grams, Fat: 39.14 grams, Carbs: 23.28 grams

6. Paprika Lamb Chops

Preparation Time 10 minutes

Cooking Time: 15 minutes

Servings: 4

Ingredients:

- 2 lamb racks, cut into chops
- Salt and pepper to taste
- 3 tablespoons paprika
- ¾ cup cumin powder
- 1 teaspoon chili powder

Directions:

- Take a bowl and add paprika, cumin, chili, salt, pepper, and stir.
- Add lamb chops and rub the mixture
- Heat grill over medium-temperature and add lamb chops, cook for 5 minutes
- Flip and cook for 5 minutes more, flip again.

- Cook for 2 minutes, flip and cook for 2 minutes more. Serve and enjoy

Nutrition: Calories: 200, Fat: 5 grams, Carbohydrates: 4 grams, Protein: 8 grams

7. Delicious Turkey Wrap

Preparation Time: 10 minutes

Cooking Time: 10 minutes

Servings: 6

Ingredients:

- 1 and a ¼ pounds of ground turkey, lean
- 4 green onions, minced
- 1 tablespoon of olive oil
- 1 garlic clove, minced
- 2 teaspoon of chili paste
- 8ounces water chestnut, diced
- 3 tablespoon of hoisin sauce
- 2 tablespoon of coconut amino
- 1 tablespoon of rice vinegar
- 12 butter lettuce leaves
- 1/8 teaspoon of salt

Directions:

- Take a pan and place it over medium heat, add turkey and garlic to the pan

- Heat for 6 minutes until cooked

- Take a bowl and transfer turkey to the bowl

- Add onions and water chestnuts

- Stir in hoisin sauce, coconut amino, vinegar, and chili paste

- Toss well and transfer the mix to lettuce leaves. Serve and enjoy.

Nutrition: Calories: 162, Fat: 4 grams, Carbohydrates: 7 grams, Protein: 23 grams

8. Bacon and Chicken Garlic Wrap

Preparation Time 15 minutes

Cooking Time: 10 minutes

Servings: 4

Ingredients:

- 1 chicken fillet, cut into small cubes
- 8-9 thin slices bacon, cut to fit cubes
- 6 garlic cloves, minced

Directions:

- Preheat your oven to 400 degrees F
- Line a baking tray with aluminum foil
- Add minced garlic to a bowl and rub each chicken piece with it
- Wrap bacon piece around each garlic chicken bite
- Secure with toothpick
- Transfer bites to the baking sheet, keeping a little bit of space between them

- Bake for about 15-20 minutes until crispy. Serve and enjoy

Nutrition: Calories: 260, Fat: 19 grams, Carbohydrates: 5 grams, Protein: 22 grams

9. Pumpkin Pancakes

Preparation Time: 10 minutes

Cooking Time: 15 minutes

Servings: 6

Ingredients:

- 3 Large eggs- Separate the egg whites for use
- 2/3 cups of organic oats
- 6 ounces pumpkin puree
- 1 scoop of collagen peptides
- 1 teaspoon stevia powder
- ½ teaspoon cinnamon
- Cooking spray

Directions:

- Blend all the ingredients together to a smooth mixture.
- Apply the cooking spray to the pan to coat it properly.

- Pour a part of the batter to the pan and let it coat the pan properly

- Wait till the edges of the pancake brown up a little bit

- Flip it over and cook from the other side

- You can serve it with fruits.

Nutrition: Calories: 70, Carbs: 16 grams, Fat: 3 grams, Protein: 3 grams

10. Cherry Smoothie Bowl

Preparation Time: 15 minutes

Cooking Time: 0 minute

Servings: 1

Ingredients:

- Soak the organic rolled oats in half a cup of unsweetened almond milk
- ½ cup of organic rolled oats
- ½ cup almond milk-unsweetened
- 1 tablespoon Chia seeds
- 1 teaspoon Help seeds
- 2 teaspoons almonds sliced
- 1 tablespoon almond butter
- 1 teaspoon vanilla extract
- ½ cup berries-fresh
- 1 cup Cherries- Frozen
- 1 cup plain Greek yogurt

Directions:

- Prepare a smooth blend of soaked oats, frozen cherries, yogurt, chia seeds, almond butter, and vanilla extract. Pour the mixture into two bowls.

- To each bowl, add the equal parts of hemp seeds, sliced almonds, and fresh cherries.

Nutrition: Calories: 130, Carbs: 32 grams, Fat: 0 gram, Protein: 1 gram

Main Meals Recipe

1. Falafel and Tahini Sauce

Preparation Time: 10 minutes

Cooking Time: 10 minutes

Servings: 2

Ingredients:

- ½ tablespoon ground coriander
- 1 teaspoon kosher salt
- 1 tablespoon ground cumin
- 1 cup raw cauliflower, pureed
- 2 large eggs
- 3 tablespoons coconut flour
- 1 clove garlic, minced
- ½ teaspoon cayenne pepper
- ½ cup ground slivered almonds
- 2 tablespoons fresh parsley, chopped

Tahini sauce:

- 1 tablespoon lemon juice
- 1 clove garlic, minced
- 2 tablespoons tahini paste
- 3 tablespoons water
- ½ teaspoon kosher salt, more to taste if desired

Directions:

- For the cauliflower, you should end up with a cup of the puree. It takes about 1 medium head (florets only) to get that much. First, chop it up with a knife, then add it to a food processor or magic bullet and pulse until it's blended but still has a grainy texture.
- You can grind the almonds in a similar manner – just don't over grind them, you want the texture.
- Combine the ground cauliflower and ground almonds in a medium bowl. Add the rest of the ingredients and stir until well blended.
- Heat a half and half mix of olive and grape seed (or any other light oil) oil until sizzling. While it's

heating, form the mix into 8 three-inch patties that are about the thickness of a hockey puck.

- Fry them four at a time until browned on one side and then flip and cook the other side. Resist the urge to flip too soon – you should see the edges turning brown before you attempt it – maybe 4 minutes or so per side. Remove to a plate lined with a paper towel to drain any excess oil.

- Serve with tahini sauce, and a tomato & parsley garnish if desired.

Tahini sauce: Blend all ingredients in a bowl. Thin with more water if you like a lighter consistency.

Nutrition: Calories: 281, Fat: 24 grams, Carbohydrates: 5 grams, Protein: 8 grams

2. Butternut Squash Risotto

Preparation Time: 10 minutes

Cooking Time: 15 minutes

Servings: 4

Ingredients:

- Butter- 3 tablespoons
- Minced sage- 2 tablespoons
- Black pepper, ground up- 1/4 teaspoon
- Minced rosemary- 1 teaspoon
- Salt- 1 teaspoon
- Dry sherry- ½ cup
- Riced cauliflower- 4 cups
- Butternut squash, cooked and mashed- ½ cup
- Parmesan cheese, grated - ½ cup
- Mascarpone cheese- ½ cup
- Grated nutmeg- 1/8 teaspoon
- Minced garlic- 1 teaspoon

Directions:

- Melt your butter inside of a large frying pan turned to a medium level of heat.

- Add your rosemary, your sage, and the garlic. Cook this for about one minute or until this mixture begins to become fragrant.

- Add in the cauliflower rice, the pepper and salt and the mashed squash. Cook this for three minutes. You will know it is ready for the next step when cauliflower is starting to soften up for you.

- Add in your sherry and cook this for an additional six minutes, or until the majority of the liquid is absorbed into the rice, or when the cauliflower is much softer.

- Stir in the mascarpone cheese, the Parmesan cheese, as well as the nutmeg (grated).

- Cook all of this on a medium heat level, being sure to stir it occasionally and do this until the cheese has melted and the risotto has gotten creamy. This will take around four to five minutes.

- Taste the risotto and add more pepper and salt to season if you wish.

- Remove your pan from the burner and garnish your risotto with more of the herbs as well as some grated parmesan. Serve and enjoy

Nutrition: Calories: 337, Fat: 25 grams, Carbohydrates: 9 grams, Fiber: 3 grams, Protein: 8 grams

3. Coated Cauliflower Head

Preparation Time: 10 minutes

Cooking Time: 40 minutes

Servings: 6

Ingredients:

- 2pounds cauliflower head
- 3 tablespoons olive oil
- 1 tablespoon butter, softened
- 1 teaspoon ground coriander
- 1 teaspoon salt
- 1 egg, whisked
- 1 teaspoon dried cilantro
- 1 teaspoon dried oregano
- 1 teaspoon tahini paste

Directions:

- Trim cauliflower head if needed.
- Preheat oven to 350F.

- In the mixing bowl, mix up together olive oil, softened butter, ground coriander, salt, whisked egg, dried cilantro, dried oregano, and tahini paste.

- Then brush the cauliflower head with this mixture generously and transfer in the tray.

- Bake the cauliflower head for 40 minutes.

- Brush it with the remaining oil mixture every 10 minutes.

Nutrition: Calories: 136, Protein: 4.43 grams, Fat: 10.71 grams, Carbohydrates: 7.8 grams

4. Cauliflower Crust Pizza

Preparation Time: 20 minutes

Cooking Time: 42 minutes

Servings: 2

Ingredients:

For Crust:

- 1 small head cauliflower, cut into florets
- 2 large organic eggs, beaten lightly
- ½ teaspoon dried oregano
- ½ teaspoon garlic powder
- Ground black pepper, as required

For Topping:

- ½ cup sugar-free pizza sauce
- ¾ cup mozzarella cheese, shredded
- ¼ cup black olives, pitted and sliced
- 2 tablespoons Parmesan cheese, grated

Directions:

- Preheat your oven to 4000 F (2000 C).

- Line a baking sheet with a lightly greased parchment paper.

- Add the cauliflower in a food processor and pulse until a rice-like texture is achieved.

- In a bowl, add the cauliflower rice, eggs, oregano, garlic powder, and black pepper and mix until well combined.

- Place the cauliflower the mixture in the center of the prepared baking sheet and with a spatula, press into a 13-inch thin circle.

- Bake for 40 minutes or until golden brown.

- Remove the baking sheet from the oven. Now, set the oven to broiler on high.

- Place the tomato sauce on top of the pizza crust and with a spatula, spread evenly and sprinkle with olives, followed by the cheeses.

- Broil for about 1-2 minutes or until the cheese is bubbly and browned.

- Remove from oven and with a pizza cutter, cut the pizza into equal-sized triangles.

- Serve hot.

Nutrition: Calories: 119 Fat: 6.6 grams, Carbohydrates: 8.6 grams, Fiber: 3.4 grams, Protein: 8.3 grams

5. Cabbage Casserole

Preparation Time: 15 minutes

Cooking Time: 30 minutes

Servings: 2

Ingredients:

- ½ head cabbage
- 2 scallions, chopped
- 4 tablespoons unsalted butter
- 2 ounces cream cheese, softened
- ¼ cup Parmesan cheese, grated
- ¼ cup fresh cream
- ½ teaspoon Dijon mustard
- 2 tablespoons fresh parsley, chopped
- Salt and ground black pepper, as required

Directions:

- Preheat your oven to 3500 F (1800 C).

- Cut the cabbage head into half, lengthwise. Then cut into 4 equal-sized wedges.

- In a pan of boiling water, add cabbage wedges and cook, covered for about 5 minutes.

- Drain well and arrange cabbage wedges into a small baking dish.

- In a small pan, melt butter and sauté onions for about 5 minutes.

- Add the remaining ingredients and stir to combine.

- Remove from the heat and immediately, place the cheese mixture over cabbage wedges evenly.

- Bake for about 20 minutes.

- Remove from the oven and let it cool for about 5 minutes before serving.

- Cut into 3 equal-sized portions and serve.

Nutrition: Calories: 273, Fat: 24.8 grams, Carbohydrates: 9 grams, Fiber: 3.4 grams, Protein: 6.2 grams

6. Salmon with Salsa

Preparation Time: 15 minutes

Cooking Time: 8 minutes

Servings: 2

Ingredients:

For Salsa:

- 1 small tomato, chopped
- 2 tablespoons red onion, chopped finely
- ¼ cup fresh cilantro, chopped finely
- 1 tablespoon jalapeño pepper, seeded and minced finely
- 1 garlic clove, minced finely
- Salt and ground black pepper, as required

For Salmon:

- 4 (5-ounces) (1-inch thick) salmon fillets
- 3 tablespoons butter
- 1 tablespoon fresh rosemary leaves, chopped

- 1 tablespoon fresh lemon juice

Directions:

- For salsa: Add all ingredients in a bowl and gently, stir to combine. With a plastic wrap, cover the bowl and refrigerate before serving.

- For salmon: season each salmon fillet with salt and black pepper generously. In a large skillet, melt butter over medium-high. Place the salmon fillets, skins side up and cook for about 4 minutes. Carefully change the side of each salmon fillet and cook for about 4 minutes more. Stir in the rosemary and lemon juice and remove from the heat. Divide the salsa onto serving plates evenly. To each plate with 1 salmon fillet and serve.

Nutrition: Calories: 481, Fat: 37.2 grams, Carbohydrates: 11 grams, Fiber: 7.6 grams, Protein: 29.9 grams

7. Zucchini Avocado Carpaccio

Preparation Time: 10 minutes

Cooking Time: 0 minute

Servings: 2

Ingredients:

- 3 Cups thinly sliced zucchini
- 1 Thinly sliced ripe avocado
- 1 tablespoon freshly squeezed lemon juice
- 1 tablespoon Extra-virgin olive oil
- ¼ tablespoon finely grated lemon zest
- ½ teaspoon freshly ground black pepper
- 1 ounce Sliced and chopped almonds
- Sea salt to taste

Directions:

- Mix the lemon juice with the lemon zest in a bowl.
- Add in the olive oil along with black pepper and sea salt.

- Thinly slice the zucchini and avocado on a plate.

- Set the avocado and zucchini and on a plate in an overlapping manner.

- Now drizzle the lemon juice mixture over the salad.

- Top the salad with the finely chopped almonds.

Nutrition: Calories: 81, Carbs: 5 grams, Fat: 6 grams, Protein: 3 grams

8. Chipotle Chicken Chowder

Preparation Time: 10 minutes

Cooking Time: 25 minutes

Servings: 2

Ingredients:

- 16 ounces Boneless, skinless, fully cooked chicken breast meat
- 3 cups Organic chicken broth
- 3 cups Coconut Milk
- 6 tablespoons Tapioca flour
- 2 tablespoons Extra-virgin olive oil
- 2 teaspoons Ground Cumin
- 7 ounces chopped green bell pepper
- 7 ounces chopped red pepper
- 7 ounces chopped white onion
- 3 Chipotle peppers in adobo sauce
- 1 Cup Water

- Spring onions for garnishing

Directions:

- Over medium heat, place your thick base saucepan and add extra-virgin olive oil.

- Add the vegetables like onion and all bell peppers along with cumin. Stir the mix thoroughly so that everything gets mixed. Cook it for a couple of minutes while stirring it occasionally.

- Add the chicken broth, water, and chipotle.

- Always remain careful of the quantity of chipotle you add. If you don't like it too hot, be careful with the quantity.

- Bring the contents to a boil.

- Reduce the heat once the mixture has come to a boil.

- Cover the saucepan and let it simmer for good 8-10 minutes.

- Add the chicken breasts.

- Prepare the tapioca flour mixture in a separate bowl.

- To make this, take the flour in a bowl and add 2/3 cup of coconut milk. Blend the mixture properly. Ensure that there are no lumps.

- Now, add this mixture to the broth in the saucepan and let it also come to a boil.

- Allow it boil for a few minutes and then add the remaining coconut milk to the broth.

- Over medium heat, continue cooking the broth for a few more minutes. Keep stirring the broth at regular intervals.

- Ensure that the soup is thick and bubbly.

- After a few minutes, transfer the soup into a bowl and garnish with chopped green onion.

Nutrition: Calories: 140, Carbs: 22 grams, Fat: 3 grams, Protein: 6 grams

9. Grilled Salmon with Avocado Salsa

Preparation Time: 15 minutes

Cooking Time: 25 minutes

Servings: 1

Ingredients:

- 16 ounces Salmon
- 1 Avocado-Sliced
- ½ Red Onion-Sliced
- 1 tablespoon Olive Oil
- ½ teaspoon Paprika Powder
- ½ teaspoon Ground Cumin
- ½ teaspoon Black Pepper
- 1/4 teaspoon Chili Powder
- Fresh Cilantro- Chopped
- 4 tablespoons Lime Juice
- Salt to taste

Directions:

- For the seasoning mix, add the chopped onions, paprika, chili powder, cumin, olive oil, and salt in a mixing bowl.

- Coat the salmon properly with the prepared mix

- Keep it in the refrigerator for at least 45 minutes

- In a separate bowl, add the avocado, onion, cilantro, and lime juice, salt. Let it cool in the fridge for a while.

- Grill the salmon from both sides.

- Eat the salmon with avocado salsa on the side.

Nutrition: Calories: 232, Carbs: 18 grams, Fat: 5 grams, Protein: 29 grams

10. Thai Tofu Curry

Preparation Time: 15 minutes

Cooking Time: 30 minutes

Servings: 2

Ingredients:

- 7 ounces Tofu- Small chunks
- 2 ounces Mangetout
- 2 ounces Baby corn- Cut in small pieces
- 1 Green chili- chopped
- 2 Shallots-Chopped
- 2 Lime leaves
- 1 Aubergine
- ½ Green pepper- thinly sliced
- 1/3 cup of lime juice
- ½ teaspoon sesame oil
- 1 teaspoon soy sauce
- 2 tablespoons green curry Thai paste

- 2 ounces vegetable stock
- 7 ounces Coconut milk
- Lime wedges for serving
- 6 ounces Long-grain Basmati rice for serving
- Chopped coriander for garnishing

Directions:

- Take a large skillet with deep sides.
- Begin by frying the shallots on medium heat for about 5 minutes.
- Add the salt as it would speed up the cooking.
- Ensure that the shallots are translucent.
- Toss in the chili and continue frying for another minute.
- You'll see the color of the shallots changing. It would be time to add the curry paste.
- Continue frying for another minute.
- Now, add the coconut milk and the Thai sauce.
- Let the mixture come to a boil.

- Once the mixture has started to boil, reduce the heat and let it simmer for another 5 minutes.

- Add the aubergine and the lime leaves. Let it cook for another 10 minutes.

- After this, add tofu and green pepper to the curry.

- Take off the lid and let it cook for 5 more minutes.

- Finally, add the mange tout, baby corn, and lime juice.

- In a separate vessel, cook your rice.

- Sprinkle coriander on the top and put the lime wedge on the side.

- Serve it hot with rice.

Nutrition: Calories: 146, Carbs: 10 grams, Fat: 8 grams, Protein: 10 grams,

Snacks Recipe

1. Roasted Brussels sprouts With Pecans and Gorgonzola

Preparation Time: 10 minutes

Cooking Time: 35 minutes

Servings: 4

Ingredients:

- Brussels Sprouts, fresh- 1 pound
- Pecans, chopped- ¼ cup
- Olive oil- 1 tablespoon
- Extra olive oil to oil the baking tray
- Pepper and salt for tasting
- Gorgonzola cheese- ¼ cup (If you prefer not to use the Gorgonzola cheese, you can toss the Brussels sprouts when hot, with 2 tablespoons of butter instead.

Directions:

- Warm the oven to 350 degrees Fahrenheit or 175 Celsius.

- Rub a large pan or any vessel you wish to use with a little bit of olive oil. You can use a paper towel or a pastry brush.

- Cut off the ends of the Brussels sprouts if you need to and then cut then in a lengthwise direction into halves. (Fear not if a few of the leaves come off of them, some may become deliciously crunchy during cooking)

- Chop up all of the pecans using a knife and then measure them for the amount.

- Put your Brussels sprouts as well as the sliced pecans inside a bowl, and cover them all with some olive oil, pepper, and salt (be generous).

- Arrange all of your pecans and Brussels sprouts onto your roasting pan in a single layer

- Roast this for 30 to 35 minutes, or when they become tender and can be pierced with a fork easily. Stir during cooking if you wish to get a more even browning.

- Once cooked, toss them with the Gorgonzola Cheese (or butter) before you serve them. Serve them hot.

Nutrition: Calories: 149, Fat: 11 grams, Carbohydrates: 10 grams, Fiber: 4 grams, Protein: 5 grams

2. Artichoke Petals Bites

Preparation Time: 10 minutes

Cooking Time: 10 minutes

Servings: 8

Ingredients:

- 8 ounces artichoke petals, boiled, drained, without salt
- ½ cup almond flour
- 4 ounces Parmesan, grated
- 2 tablespoons almond butter, melted

Directions:

- In the mixing bowl, mix up together almond flour and grated Parmesan.
- Preheat the oven to 355F.
- Dip the artichoke petals in the almond butter and then coat in the almond flour mixture.
- Place them in the tray.
- Transfer the tray in the preheated oven and cook the petals for 10 minutes.

- Chill the cooked petal bites little before serving.

Nutrition: Calories: 93, Protein: 6.54 grams, Fat: 3.72 grams, Carbohydrates: 9.08 grams

3. Stuffed Beef Loin in Sticky Sauce

Preparation Time: 15 minutes

Cooking Time: 6 minutes

Servings: 4

Ingredients:

- 1 tablespoon Erythritol
- 1 tablespoon lemon juice
- 4 tablespoons water
- 1 tablespoon butter
- ½ teaspoon tomato sauce
- ¼ teaspoon dried rosemary
- 9 ounces beef loin
- 3 ounces celery root, grated
- 3 ounces bacon, sliced
- 1 tablespoon walnuts, chopped
- ¾ teaspoon garlic, diced
- 2 teaspoons butter

- 1 tablespoon olive oil
- 1 teaspoon salt
- ½ cup of water

Directions:

- Cut the beef loin into the layer and spread it with the dried rosemary, butter, and salt. Then place over the beef loin: grated celery root, sliced bacon, walnuts, and diced garlic.
- Roll the beef loin and brush it with olive oil. Secure the meat with the help of the toothpicks. Place it in the tray and add a ½ cup of water.
- Cook the meat in the preheated to 365F oven for 40 minutes.

Meanwhile, make the sticky sauce:

- Mix up together Erythritol, lemon juice, 4 tablespoons of water, and butter.
- Preheat the mixture until it starts to boil. Then add tomato sauce and whisk it well.
- Bring the sauce to boil and remove from the heat.
- When the beef loin is cooked, remove it from the oven and brush with the cooked sticky sauce very generously.

- Slice the beef roll and sprinkle with the remaining sauce.

Nutrition: Calories: 321, Protein: 18.35 grams, Fat: 26.68 grams, Carbohydrates: 2.75 grams

4. Eggplant Fries

Preparation Time 10 minutes

Cooking Time: 15 minutes

Servings: 8

Ingredients:

- 2 eggs
- 2 cups almond flour
- 2 tablespoons coconut oil, spray
- 2 eggplant, peeled and cut thinly
- Salt and pepper

Directions:

- Preheat your oven to 400 degrees Fahrenheit
- Take a bowl and mix with salt and black pepper in it
- Take another bowl and beat eggs until frothy
- Dip the eggplant pieces into eggs
- Then coat them with flour mixture

- Add another layer of flour and egg

- Then, take a baking sheet and grease with coconut oil on top

- Bake for about 15 minutes

- Serve and enjoy.

Nutrition Calories: 212, Fat: 15.8 grams, Carbohydrates: 12.1 grams, Protein: 8.6 grams

5. Parmesan Crisps

Preparation Time 5 minutes

Cooking Time: 25 minutes

Servings: 8

Ingredients:

- 1 teaspoon butter
- 8 ounces parmesan cheese, full fat and shredded

Directions:

- Preheat your oven to 400 degrees F
- Put parchment paper on a baking sheet and grease with butter
- Spoon parmesan into 8 mounds, spreading them apart evenly
- Flatten them
- Bake for 5 minutes until browned
- Let them cool
- Serve and enjoy.

Nutrition: Calories: 133, Fat: 11 grams, Carbohydrates: 1gram, Protein: 11 grams

6. Roasted Broccoli

Preparation Time 5 minutes

Cooking Time: 20 minutes

Servings: 4

Ingredients:

- 4 cups broccoli florets
- 1 tablespoon olive oil
- Salt and pepper to taste

Directions:

- Preheat your oven to 400 degrees F
- Add broccoli in a zip bag alongside oil and shake until coated
- Add seasoning and shake again
- Spread broccoli out on the baking sheet, bake for 20 minutes
- Let it cool and serve.

Nutrition: Calories: 62, Fat: 4 grams, Carbohydrates: 4 grams, Protein: 4 grams

7. Almond Flour Muffins

Preparation Time: 15 minutes

Cooking Time: 30 minutes

Servings: 8

Ingredients:

- 1/3 cup of pumpkin puree
- 3 eggs
- 2 tablespoons agave nectar
- 2 tablespoons coconut oil
- 1 teaspoon vanilla extract
- 1 teaspoon white vinegar
- 1 cup chopped fruits
- 1 teaspoon baking soda
- ½ teaspoon salt

Directions:

- Preheat the oven to 350°F.
- Line the muffin tin with paper liners

- In the first mixing bowl, whisk the almond flour, salt, and baking soda.

- In the second mixing bowl, whisk the pumpkin puree, eggs, coconut oil, agave nectar, vanilla extract, and vinegar.

- Now add this puree mix of the second bowl to the first bowl and blend everything well.

- Add the chopped fruits to the blend.

- Pour the mixture to the muffin cups in your pan.

- Bake for 15-20 minutes. Ensure that the contents have set in the center, and a golden brown lining has started to appear at the edges.

- Transfer the muffins to a cooling rack and let it cool completely.

Nutrition: Calories: 75, Carbs: 4 grams, Fat: 6 grams, Protein: 0 gram

8. Squash Bites

Preparation Time: 10 minutes

Cooking Time: 40 minutes

Servings: 4

Ingredients:

- 10 ounces of turkey meat, cooked, sliced
- 2 pounds butternut squash, cubed
- 1 teaspoon chili powder
- 1 teaspoon garlic powder
- 1 teaspoon sweet paprika
- Black pepper to taste

Directions:

- In a bowl, mix butternut squash cubes with chili powder, black pepper, garlic powder and paprika and toss to coat.
- Wrap squash pieces in turkey slices, place them all on a lined baking sheet, place in the oven at 350 degrees F, bake for 20 minutes, flip and bake for 20 minutes more.

- Arrange squash bites on a platter and serve. Enjoy

Nutrition: Calories 223, Fat 3.8 grams, Fiber 4.5 grams, Carbs 26.5 grams, Protein 23 grams

9. Zucchini Chips

Preparation Time: 10 minutes

Cooking Time: 12 minutes

Servings: 4

Ingredients:

- 1 zucchini, thinly sliced
- A pinch of sea salt
- Black pepper to taste
- 1 teaspoon thyme, dried
- 1 egg
- 1 teaspoon garlic powder
- 1 cup almond flour

Directions:

- In a bowl, whisk the egg with a pinch of salt.
- Put the flour in another bowl and mix it with thyme, black pepper, and garlic powder.
- Dredge zucchini slices in the egg mix and then in flour.

- Arrange chips on a lined baking sheet, place in the oven at 450 degrees F and bake for 6 minutes on each side,

- Serve the zucchini chips as a snack. Enjoy.

Nutrition: Calories: 106, Fat: 8.2 grams, Carbs: 5.2 grams, Protein: 5.1 grams, Fiber 2.1 grams

10.   Pepperoni Bites

Preparation Time: 5 minutes

Cooking Time: 10 minutes

Servings: 24 pieces

Ingredients:

- 1/3 cup tomatoes, chopped
- ½ cup bell peppers, mixed and chopped
- 24 pepperoni slices
- ½ cup tomato sauce
- 4 ounces almond cheese, cubed
- 2 tablespoons basil, chopped
- Black pepper to taste

Directions:

- Divide pepperoni slices into a muffin tray.
- Divide tomato and bell pepper pieces into the pepperoni cups.
- Also divide the tomato sauce, basil and almond cheese cubes, sprinkle black pepper at the end,

place cups in the oven at 400 degrees F and bake for 10 minutes.

- Arrange the pepperoni bites on a platter and serve.

Nutrition: Calories 59, Fat 4.5 grams, Fiber 0.1 gram, Carbs 2 grams, Protein 2.5 grams

Conclusion

If this has taught you anything, the hope is that it has taught you how many variables are involved when it comes to health and wellness. This aimed to share with you the plethora of options that are available to you when it comes to intermittent fasting and autophagy, as well as how to induce it within the cells of your body in order to achieve desired results and outcomes.

Think back on the many options that were laid out for you in this book involving diet options and specific foods that have the ability to induce autophagy in the brain. It is your job now to decide which of these foods or supplements to include in your life and to practice a sort of trial and error, noting which ones make you feel great and which ones you prefer to go without. With all of this information, you can decide which ways fit best with your specific lifestyle and your preferences.

As you can see, there are many different ways to optimize autophagy. The way or ways that you choose will be highly dependent on you as an individual. You may want to approach this by trying one and being open to changing methods if it does not work as well as you would like. You may want to try a combination of methods in order to get the best results. The key is to be flexible and be open to change, as nobody knows how their body will react to changes in diet and exercise.

In anything new that we try, there is a chance that we may fall off track. Fasting or following a new diet plan is no different. The focus should not be on the fact that you fell off but on how you decide to come back and approach it again. You need not give up altogether if you have a day or two where you did not accomplish your full fast. You just need to re-examine your plan and approach it in a different way. Maybe your fasting period was too long for your first try. Maybe your fasting and eating windows did not match up with your sleep-wake cycle as well as they could have. Any of these factors can be adjusted to better suit your lifestyle needs and make fasting or a specific diet work for you. With the human body, there is never a right or a wrong way to approach anything; there is only a multitude of different ways and some that will be better for your specific body and mind than others. Being open to trying different variations and adjusting your plan as you go can be the difference between success and decided to give up.

If you fall off track, scale your plan back a little bit and try it again. If you are worried that you are not doing enough, begin with the scaled-back plan and get used to this first. You can always increase your fasting times later on once you know you are completely comfortable with a shorter fasting time.

As you can see, there are numerous benefits that come with employing an intermittent fasting diet. I promised you that within these pages you would find out why your body reacts differently to diet programs and how you can deal with it, and that I would provide you with specific examples of intermittent fasting programs that were designed with your sex and age in mind. After reading this, you now have this information and much, much more! You are fully equipped to begin changing your life with programs designed specifically for you, and I hope that you feel empowered to do so!

The main takeaway is that there are many options for women over the age of 50 to take control of their weight loss strategies, without having to turn to methods designed for men or people in their twenties. Further, taking control of your health and playing an active role in your disease risk reduction is not as difficult as it sounds. I hope that after reading this, you have a new understanding of what you can do and how your body will react given your age and sex.

As you take all of this information forth with you, it may seem overwhelming to begin applying this into your own life. Remember, life is a process, and you do not need to expect perfection from yourself. By reading this, you are already on your way to changing your life.

Did you enjoy this book?

If you enjoyed this book, it would be awesome if you could leave a quick review on Amazon. Your feedback is much appreciated and I would love to hear from you.

<u>Leave a Review on Amazon</u>

Thanks so much!!

More books by Geena Moore:

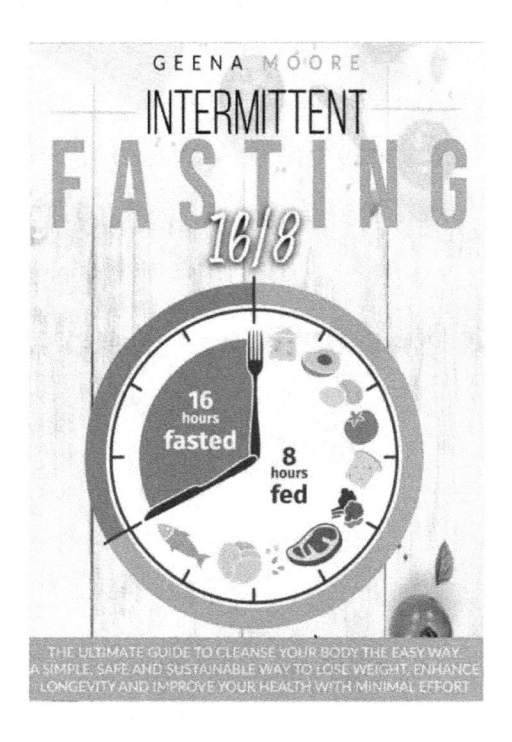

Intermittent Fasting 16/8: The Ultimate Guide To Cleanse Your Body The Easy Way. A Simple, Safe and Sustainable Way to Lose Weight, Enhance Longevity and Improve Your Health with Minimal Effort. (Link)

More books by Geena Moore:

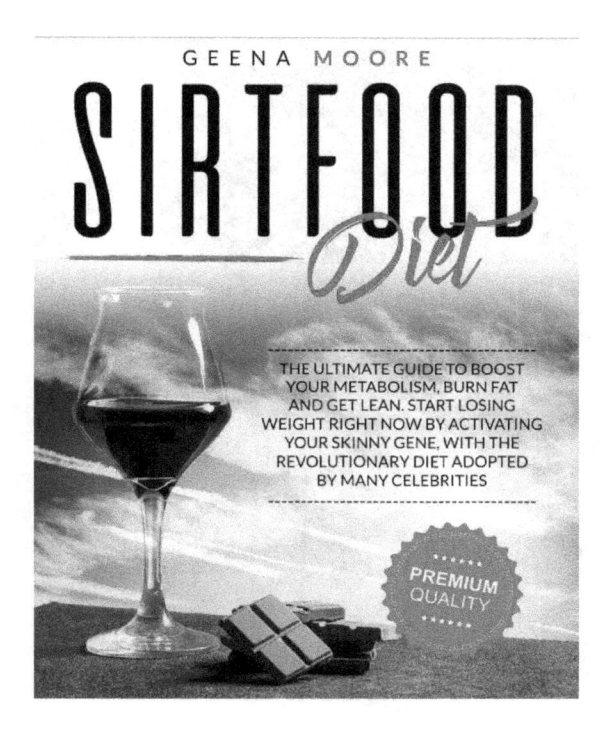

Sirtfood Diet: The Ultimate Guide to Boost YOUR Metabolism, Burn Fat and Get Lean. Start Losing Weight RIGHT NOW by Activating Your Skinny Gene with the Revolutionary Diet Adopted by Many Celebrities. (Link)

More books by Geena Moore:

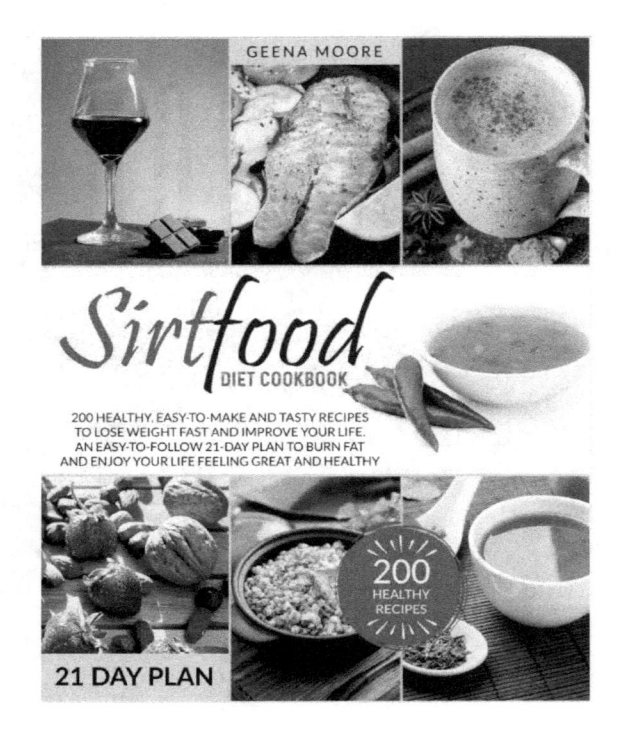

Sirtfood Diet Cookbook: 200 Healthy, Easy-To-Make and Tasty Recipes to Lose Weight Fast and Improve YOUR Life. An Easy-To-Follow 21-Day Plan to Burn Fat and Enjoy YOUR Life Feeling Great and Healthy. (Link)

CPSIA information can be obtained
at www.ICGtesting.com
Printed in the USA
BVHW041035011220
594600BV00007B/183